Interspersed with narratives from her hospital record, Gray encodes a journey through the biopsychology of identity—physical, spiritual, artistic.

These poems brilliantly enact Rimbaud's meme, "Je est un autre": the claim that "I" is an "other" as the starting point for true artistic originality. In Gray, the case is forced. The other is a brain tumor growing in her falx, a curved blade of tissue that partitions the two hemispheres; the tumor that divides her. First, terror. The invasiveness, the foreignness, is conceived in a way perfectly concordant with the surgeon's intent: excision, "taking with it / all the family cancers / all my friends' pulmonary / failures...every malevolence...taken / to the limits of the village / and cast out". She imagines she can select the deletions "after the erasure"; and choose their replacements: "The ten wheels / Of inexhaustible ornament, / The nine nectars of inner radiance".

Inflected with Gray's decades-long study of *The Tibetan Book of the Dead*, her post-op liminal state is a kind of Bardo, the transitional state between death and rebirth where language meets its limits and otherworldly visions prepare for what is to come. But who is writing? Who survives? Now, in a volta that emerges in the book itself, the poems turn: a feeling for the tumor, for its absence, for what it had been, and meant.

. . . Only the
departing surgeons

know that behind the resealed
walls hang lily of the valley

curtains and the photo
of a soldier

above where
his bed had been)

The poet begins to worry about the tumor:

. . . How much of it

had been discarded, how much
had it overheard

Did it remember her

First the estrangement, then wonderment, and a completely alternate sensibility: Who was invasive? Who were the invaders? The tumor becomes an intimate, mysterious; a lost, loved one. "Something that desired / to be understood // heard, seen / but not touched". I, an other, irreplaceable by a bone window and a titanium plate.

Riveting, utterly original, Gray mobilizes the matter, the material, of her falx meningioma; not, as does the surgeon, to remove all vestiges, but as a poet. It has become a guiding wonderment, a new lucidity, made from fragments under a bone saw.

"What did it say, the note the tumor had been writing at its desk in the familiar dark?"

Dawn McGuire, MD
Fellow of the American Academy of Neurology
Author of the poetry collections *The Aphasia Cafe* and *American Dream with Exit Wound*

AFTER THE OPERATION

Also by Elizabeth T. Gray, Jr.:

Salient
Series | India

Translations

The Green Sea of Heaven: 80 Ghazals of Háfiz-i Shirází, 30th Anniversary Edition.
Let Us Believe in the Beginning of the Cold Season: Selected Poems of Forough Farrokhzad (1934–1967)
Wine & Prayer: Eighty Ghazals from the Díwán of Háfiz
Iran: Poems of Dissent
The Green Sea of Heaven: Fifty Ghazals from the Díwán of Háfiz

AFTER THE OPERATION

Elizabeth T. Gray, Jr.

Library of Congress Cataloging-in-Publication Data

Names: Gray, Elizabeth T. Jr., 1952– author.
Title: After the operation / Elizabeth T. Gray, Jr.
Description: New York : Four Way Books, 2025.
Identifiers: LCCN 2024035162 (print) | LCCN 2024035163 (ebook) |
ISBN 9781961897403 (trade paperback) | ISBN 9781961897410 (ebook)
Subjects: LCGFT: Poetry.
Classification: LCC PS3607.R3889 A68 2025 (print) | LCC PS3607.R3889
(ebook) | DDC 811/.6—dc23/eng/20240802
LC record available at https://lccn.loc.gov/2024035162
LC ebook record available at https://lccn.loc.gov/2024035163

This book is manufactured in the United States of America and printed on acid-free paper.

Four Way Books is a not-for-profit literary press. We are grateful for the assistance we receive from individual donors, public arts agencies, and private foundations including the New York State Council on the Arts, a state agency.

NEW YORK STATE OF OPPORTUNITY. Council on the Arts

PROUD MEMBER [clmp]

We are a proud member of the Community of Literary Magazines and Presses.

To my husband, Chip, and my boys, Sam and William, for their warm and sustaining care

To the flocks of friends who appeared in the winter sky

To John G. Golfinos, MD, Jessica Schafrick, NP, and the entire team at NYU Langone's Department of Neurosurgery for their competence, professionalism, and sense of humor

In memory of
my friends Robert Riskind and Marguerite Yates,
my colleague Terry Barnett, and
my first cousin Morris Gray,
whose brain tumors gave no quarter

After the operation, her mind
became an uninhabited coast

When we found her she offered
us bone fragment and sea-

weathered wood, asking
what they meant

What looked like someone with her
was a tall stone that leaned in

as if suddenly understood
"It was all shatter

and thoroughfare," she said
and pointed to the wind

(After the operation,

intact abandoned
its nouns, the idea

itself fell
apart and was

last seen somewhere
in an enamel

bowl in pieces
next to a bone saw)

Physician's Progress Notes
October 27, 2020

Elizabeth Gray is a 68-year-old corporate consultant. An MRI in 2014 was performed and unexpectedly showed an anterior skull base meningioma at the planum sphenoidale. The tumor has gradually increased in size since that time. We had a long discussion with her considering the options for treatment. We discussed that her alternatives include continued watchful waiting versus surgical resection, versus Gamma Knife radiosurgery. I told her that I am usually conservative with incidentally found tumors. However, she did not want to wait longer on this tumor. She wanted a definitive solution to this problem. We discussed the alternative of radiation. She favored definitive resection. Given her family history of meningiomas, and her friends' brain cancers, she expressed the certainty that she would like the tumor dealt with now before it becomes too big. We have therefore recommended surgical resection as the best option for treatment.

We discussed the risks of surgery including but not limited to coma, death, stroke, paralysis, infection, bleeding, and spinal fluid leak. Specific to this tumor in this location, we also discussed the risks of complete loss of olfaction, spinal fluid leak into the ethmoid or frontal sinus (which is small on the MRI), and damage to the frontal lobes with change in personality. We described the procedure in detail. We discussed the pre- and postoperative courses as well as discharge instructions and restrictions. We discussed the location of the incision behind her hairline and that we would likely only need to shave minimal hair. We discussed the risk of a medical complication. In summary, the risks, benefits, and alternatives to surgery were discussed with the patient. All questions were answered, and the patient expressed her full understanding. She wishes to proceed with the planned surgery and has given consent.

(They tell me it will be a right pterional resection. Of an anterior falx meningioma.

What does this mean.

The *pterion,* in the temporal fossa. Site of the convergence of important plates: the parietal bone, the temporal bone, the frontal bone, and the *greater wing* of the sphenoid bone.

A *structural landmark* for neurological access.

The weakest part of the skull.

From *pteron,* meaning *wing* or *feather.*

The precise location where trickster Hermes's wings were.

There will be what they call a *bone window.* And then titanium.)

She said,

“After the operation the tumor
will be gone, taking with it

all the family cancers
all my friends’ pulmonary

failures, their own flavors
of tumor

Mine will be
the thread cross

that will ensnare
every malevolence

in its skein of veins and then
by this superb medical team

be extracted carefully
from under my frontal lobe’s

low overhang, taken
to the limits of the village

and cast out."

January 13, 2021

(The last of *before*
was a moment before dawn filled

with pale blue beings
backlit and masked

speaking softly
in a thicket of screens

How fast it all was:
four portals

taped into my arms
and waiting

After all that wholehearted consent
I never saw them again)

Surgeon's Operative Notes
January 13, 2021

After the resection, all of the cottonoids and Telfas were removed and the tumor bed was inspected under magnification. No residual tumor was found. We felt that we had a gross total resection.

The bed was copiously irrigated to ensure hemostasis. Small bleeding points were controlled with the bipolar. The bed was then lined with surgical squares. Irrigation returned crystal clear. Hemostasis was complete. We began closure. The dural flap was then rotated back into position. The dura was re-approximated with interrupted and running sutures of 4-0 Neurolon. A central dural tack-up was placed. A layer of thin Gelfoam was placed over the dura. The bone flap was plated back into position using the Stryker microplates. The wound was irrigated several times copiously with Bacitracin irrigation. The muscle was reattached to the superior cuff and to the holes drilled at the temporal line. The muscle was closed posteriorly as well with interrupted sutures of 2-0 Vicryl. The skin was closed in two layers with 2-0 Vicryl on the galea in inverted interrupted fashion and staples on the skin.

The patient was then released from the Mayfield frame and placed back in supine position on the hospital bed. The Mayfield tongs were removed. The monitoring leads were removed and a standard neurosurgical head wrap was applied. The SSEPs and MEPs remained intact throughout the procedure. The patient was awakened, extubated, and taken to the ICU in stable condition, where she was following commands and moving all four extremities with normal power. All counts were correct.

We came upon her at dusk
in a dense forest

of monitors
draped cuffs, dangling

salines, tapes, drains
broad bandages, electrodes

We tried not to be terrified
and failed

We looked to her as we always had
We tried to tell her she looked fine

Because she could not see herself
she tried to put us at ease

We asked her how she felt, really
She was very calm (the meds)

"I was worried," she said
"but nothing has changed. Listen,

beyond the windows:
the creak of bullock carts

breaking waves, crows,
the call to prayer."

(After the operation,

there were three birds
outside on the ledge

Everyone was uncertain
what that meant

but I knew:
"This omen

is for the others,"
I said, pointing

across the volcanoes to the
cancered and the dead)

January 15, 2021

(After the operation, what they wanted
was the me they knew

“I want that too,” I said
trying to distract them

from the holes where
tent pegs had been

from the faint oryx tracks that ran
northeast between the broken

mud walls through tamarisk
toward the patient

elevators and
the nurses’ station)

(After the operation, there were birds
Birds you could see, birds you couldn't

Alighted, quiet on the bedrail
The rustling not bedsheets or leaves

but feathers: warmth offered
from beneath a wing

This profusion of blue, display of
not yet fully-understood beauty

As things settle and other parts go silent
the feathers become easier to hear)

January 18, 2021

(Journal Entry

After the operation, how it went and what happened, how it felt, how the drugs protected my brain from swelling and seizures, from itself, how visitors did or did not appear, how the pain circumambulated my skull clumsily like an underfunded amateur explorer, how people came and went among the machines, who actually was there and mattered, who was not and now doesn't, how slowly the titanium and bone got to know each other, and how the skewed world tried to reassert itself pushing reminders, recaps, and synopses—it all could be read like striations of archaic soot in ice, glyphs across the glacier's uneasy face, but from a safe distance.)

She had been brought
carefully

by skilled anesthesiologists
back into time

but after the operation the calendar
stalled

Wednesday for example
like a high-pressure system

over the Great Plains
The 19th set to continue

through February
Cold fronts of pain

After the operation, *expedition*
was much diminished as in

to the kitchen from a base camp
stocked with medication

eyeshades, Tylenol
topo maps, maybe oxygen

past the guestroom and linen
closet onto the narrow

plateau of the hall
where yesterday she said

she saw Sherpas smoking
in the lee of a low wall

(After the operation, some people
no longer were

Scenes in which they had been
gone also but, as if each were a tumor

I could point
to where they had been

Andrew for example
no longer, nor on that bridge

The tea stall where Nadia never showed
now a river)

(A nurse had told me
to sleep

Then where she had been
just woodsmoke

damp mountain air
on the river

and the sound of
a receding Jeep)

"After the operation,
I could see," she said
"those failures struggling

in the high-sided half-
filled pail to breathe
each thing

trying to
climb over the
others for air."

After the operation, the desolation
was not behind her

As when a storm has passed, bleaching the air,
and the stones are still there

"I thought," she said, "that after
being under, the erasure, the

evisceration and terror,
the acceptance of risk, of severance,

I would no longer be stalked by
familiar emaciates staggering

across the dark plain
hawking their sacks of grief."

(Out in the corridor
again the barred

owl, soundless, all
portent

For days afterward I asked
everyone to scour the room:

nothing, not even
small rinds of fur)

January 27, 2021

(They removed the staples
from the zigzagged incision that

through the tangles
of my hair ran

like an abandoned trench system
seen from the air

Where I had lost my nerves
right there was

a clearing where an AH-64 Apache
or a UH-60 Black Hawk could come in)

February 2021

(After the operation, there were gaps
into which things fell

but these were richly appointed
and rode a turquoise horse

Each opened out onto a riverbed of gravels
and braided, silt-filled waters

that could be followed
back up into the Annapurnas)

"If what really matters
remains intact," she said,

"then what do all these cries
of different kinds

cowering in corners
and scuttling

along the baseboards
want?"

(The weather radar shows bands
of advancing snow and I weep

I want white to muffle
but not cold I tell them

as black garbage bags calve
from the glacier face of this ornate and

intransigent grief onto
the sidewalk and move out to sea)

In between those that had been familiar
new months appeared

She erased or rearranged
the unanchored weeks

the possibilities like some
enormous double-hulled

disturbance pushing aside
sea ice

The new months were each
a hushed caldera of grey ash

placed among all the other
Arbitrary Demarcations

"After the operation, the enumerations
may stabilize," the doctors said

She was desperate to be rid
of what she called the Twenty-Four Ashen

Precepts, the Six Transparent
Omissions, the Eight Spokes
of Orphaned Commitments

Immediately she had
replacements: the Ten Wheels
of Inexhaustible Ornament,

the Nine Nectars of Inner Radiance

March 2021

(After the operation, friends were different:
from sparse to suddenly everywhere

undetectable in empty air
then suddenly everywhere jasmine

And those not there, had
they just been

imagined or mis-
classified, had they also

been piece by piece
by piece resected

out of that bone
window)

There remains the delicate matter
of the cache of feathers

She claims to preen each
as she had been taught

Her bird remains dead
and had been green

From wherever he is he tells her
the air will hold her up

She looks for pinfeathers
under her shaved scalp

By the door she sees a blue pile
of primaries, secondaries

She is frantic to make a wing
as his had been

We try to hold her
soothe her

Nervous drab birds
fret at the window

Wherever she points
all we can see is tin

(There were so many burials
They had happened while I couldn't pay attention

I tried to reassemble them
but as with time and my skull

there are pieces missing so I went back
to counting: the one

mother, the two cousins,
my raptor, the four friends,

the seven versions
of things will be OK

eaten away
from the extremities in)

April 2021

(The unnumbered fragments
of the inpatient days

would not fuse into narrative
How to fit in

pain and being
woken so often

Might my mended skull
be some post-Blitz brownstone

and in the street only the
departing surgeons

know that behind the resealed
walls hang lily of the valley

curtains and the photo
of a soldier

above where
his bed had been)

She fretted about the tumor
Where was it, bits of it

on slides in freezers, shipped
to other research centers

out there in the bright cold,
riven, no longer

afloat and warm
How much of it

had been discarded, how much
had it overheard

Did it remember her

May 2021

(Every morning I take
the year apart

There are always 7½ hours
of January missing

I even searched next August

Maybe those hours

had wandered there—bruised and
exhausted, in pressure

boots, stapled seams
glinting in sunlight

rattling bottles of
Oxycodone, dragging

their bafflement
across the hot sand,

gulls keeping
their distance)

(After the operation any sequence
could be easily disassembled and

out of such rich disarray
previously unimagined constellations

crowded toward me
and removed their clothes)

(Journal Entry June 14, 2021

Today I felt I was ready to read the core section of the surgeon's Operative Report:

The Brainlab frameless stereotactic system had been registered to the contours of the scalp using the surface-fitting algorithm. The correlation was excellent, within 0.8 mm in most areas. The Brainlab system was used to map the trajectory to the lesion and to map the frontal sinus. The incision was a curvilinear standard pterional incision. The incision was then clipped, prepped, draped in the usual aseptic fashion. The skin incision was made with the #10 blade. The incision was carried down to bone superiorly and the temporalis muscle inferiorly. The Bovie electrocautery was used to divide the temporalis. We dissected in the inter fascial plane in order to fully free up the temporalis muscle. The temporalis was then taken off the orbital rim slightly. The temporalis was then divided posteriorly with the Bovie and then superiorly. A cuff was left superiorly and additional holes were drilled at the superior temporal line. The temporalis muscle was then elevated off the bone with the Bovie. The muscle was retracted inferiorly with fish hooks while the skin flap was retracted anteriorly with fish hooks.

The Brainlab was now used to map out the contours of the tumor and plan the craniotomy contours. A single burr hole was made inferiorly with the Acu-Cut perforator and two burr holes were made superiorly at the temporal line. The dura was freed up with the #3 Penfield dissector. The Midas Rex craniotome was then used to turn the pterional bone flap with a frontal extension and small temporal exposure. The bone flap was elevated off the underlying dura which was intact. Now that the whole of the sealed doorway was laid bare, various seal impressions bearing the cartouche of the patient were discernible. After clearing the rest of the descending passage we came upon a second sealed doorway, which was almost the exact replica of the first. It bore similar seal impressions. Feverishly we cleared away the remaining last scraps of rubbish on the floor of the passage before the doorway, until we had only the clean sealed doorway before us, in which, after making preliminary notes, we made a tiny breach in the top left corner to see what was beyond.

It was some time before one could see but as soon as one's eyes became accustomed to the glimmer of light the interior of the chamber gradually loomed before one, with its strange and wonderful medley of extraordinary and beautiful objects heaped upon one another: two strange ebony-black effigies of a King, gold sandalled, bearing staff and mace; gilded couches in strange forms, lion-headed, Hathor-headed; exquisitely painted, inlaid, and ornamental caskets; alabaster vases; a lovely lotiform wishing-cup in translucent alabaster; and, lastly a confusion of overturned parts of chariots glinting with gold. Under the lobular overhang the tumor was of yellow crystalline sandstone, slightly tinted, having the four goddesses Isis, Nephthys, Neith, and Selkit in gold at each corner, their winged arms outstretched protecting it.)

(They had built a virtual three-
dimensional model, wielded

cranial drill, scalpel
to burrow carefully, deliberately

through layers
of dura sealed

with talismans, cartouches into
my never-violated dark

The tumor has been carefully removed
The chamber has been resealed

The embalmed tumor
floats somewhere in a canopic jar

The jar has the head of a hawk
The crocodile slips away

The jackal stands down
The ibis writes it all up

The feather on the scale
is blue

“Weep for Neith, Nephthys,
Selkit, Isis,” I told them,

“graceful, bereft
together in the familiar dark

golden arms outstretched
protecting where it had always been.”)

(What had been fragments
started to look

whole, no longer scattered
spall but chronicles

narratives in their own right
into which I dove, returning

to the surface with treasure:
a phrase, leaf, pearls

a harvest of shards, the task
not to reassemble

but to embrace each flake:
hierophany in an edge

Skull as broken ceramic bowl mended
as by the Japanese *kintsugi* masters

with rare things:
skill, precious metal, ceremony

Is there a *hanko* seal somewhere
under my hair that says

John G. Golfinos, MD
of New York

In her Sixty-Eighth Year)

July 2021

Eventually it became summer

We tried to move on
and were wrong

We pointed to the gulls suspended
above the sunlit undulant sea

and reminded her of the good
the fine things she had once said

that had changed us
Our remindings were a song

we thought good
and wrote down

"Nothing is back,"
she said

After the operation
went on and on

July 20, 2021

(It was definitely summer
The ice retreated

The topography of my skull
was dramatically altered:

a shallow depression where the bone window was
Unstable geology, bone

tectonics trying to configure themselves
as before and failing

New scans reveal an absence
of tumor, the presence

of nothing, the brainfolds closing in
reluctantly, as one holds a space open

for the lost child

Somewhere on the wall

of my skull are there ochre
outlines of the surgeon's

hand, or of aurochs, leopards, hawks, all
my Protectors when I was under)

(On the six-month post-op scans
beneath clefts and folds

I could see the clearing by the river
where the tumor had been:

woodsmoke through trees
a temple bell, cormorants

and one fishing boat among reeds

The artist puts down his brush

North of the Great Wall fighting continues
The Emperor is hard-pressed)

Her brain as seafloor
An occluded topography:

eloquent fissures, ridges, reconfigured
archipelagos of *silent* tissue

whose role the neuroscientists still don't
entirely understand—

the relationship of this rocky headland
to who she is, for example

August 2021

(The terror
had been on the same ferry

It disembarked in the sun
under the wheeling gulls

It had been photoshopped out
of my birthday but there it was

on the quay, carrying
in its briefcase

how it had really been,
demanding we talk

It handed me an envelope
with its credentials: the moments

I had carefully avoided
and its list of deleted scenes)

(Or the terror came
in out of the rain—

drying its thighs
with the towel it asked for—

fed up with lurking at
the edges of how

I had been
telling the story)

September 2021

It appeared that the seasons
would keep on going

and as they turned the calderas
of her skull deepened

the brain settling still
adjusting in its own time

The green leaves, like her sense of smell
dulled and frayed

"Winter will grow back," she said
"Your tumor will not," they said

October 2021

(I see differently
I know who was really

around me, I have refined
the important rituals

and above all I am
fully fledged

The long blue primaries
when extended stretch from

horizon to
horizon)

(Beneath the dura
mater and other layered

meninges, in the thicket
of blood vessels had been

something that desired
to be understood

heard, seen
but not touched

Is there a little plaque
at the base of my anterior falx

saying what had been there
and when it had been taken away)

November 24, 2022
Thanksgiving Day

(If we met again, my tumor
and I, in the layers of another lining

what would we say to one another
Would an apology be in order)

December 2022

(Snow, an erratic plow
Another winter

No smell, no taste
also no tumor

I am foraging in soiled snow
for a way to put this

behind me)

She writes down
the Thirty Vanished Scents:

garbage, seaweed, dung fires, perfume, musk,
garlic, whiskey, bacon, woodsmoke,
old books, Chennai, grasses, dog, horse, bird, her husband,
cider, pears, low tide, cedar,
oranges, eucalyptus, pepper, thyme, onion, a storm at sea,
dry leaves, cherry blossoms, roses, clove

and the Ten Olfactory Hallucinations:

hot metal, vitamins, the future, betrayal, sulfur, counterfactuals,
intentions, departure, cognition, flight

(Journal Entry January 20, 2022

What did it say, the note the tumor had been writing at its desk in the familiar dark? When they came for it had the tumor been in the middle of something, had it sensed time was running out?

The horsemen in the courtyard, waiting. The clank of weapons and armor in the hall.

Did it look up, surprised? Did it ask for some last privilege or reprieve? Did it surrender those pages to the surgeon or tuck them into a warm, suddenly lit-up fold of wall? Did it have time?

Here is my new question:

When they come for you, when the unfamiliar roar comes, and a sudden opening, and light pours in, when what had kept you safe, what had always been, is breached, pried open, and light pours in, what do you want to have been writing then?)

February 10, 2022
Physician Progress Notes

I had the pleasure of seeing Elizabeth T. Gray, Jr. today, in a neurosurgical follow-up now 12 months after right pterional resection of an anterior falx meningioma. I am pleased to say that she is doing very well. She tells me today that she is doing well and does not have any complaints at all. She does not feel that her normal olfaction has returned. She has not noted any other changes in cognition or neurologic function. The final pathology was meningioma, WHO Grade I without any unusual features. The tumor stained positively for progesterone receptors. On examination today her speech was fluent and her vocabulary was abundant. Her cognition was intact. Extraocular movements were intact. Her face was completely symmetric. She had normal and coordinated movements in all 4 extremities with normal power. She had a normal gait. We reviewed her repeat MRI scan done today and compared it to the preoperative scan with her. I showed her the areas of the tumor resection. The scan done today shows no evidence of residual or recurrent disease. I have asked her to return to see us in a year's time. Hopefully she will have some return of olfaction between now and then. She knows to call us at any time for any new question, concerns, or symptoms.

(Months go by
Nothing recurs

No glint of helmets
No campfires anywhere

In the watchtowers
they play cards

"Too quiet,"
says the garrison commander

A sentry comes on watch
in scrubs, salutes

does another scan of the horizon
adds it to my file)

NOTES

The MRI images, as well as portions of the neurosurgeon's Progress Notes and Operative Report, are drawn from my personal medical records at NYU Langone Medical Center in New York City.

The type of thread-cross referred to on page 8 is a Tibetan *gtang mdos*, used to cage or ensnare demons and other kinds of malevolent forces. See Réne de Nebesky-Wojkowitz, *Oracles and Demons of Tibet: The Cult and Iconography of the Tibetan Protective Deities* (The Hague: Mouton, 1956. Kathmandu and Varanasi: Book Faith India, 1993, p. 369 and ff.)

Line 2 on page 18 ("Birds you could see, birds you couldn't") is an informal translation of a line from Farīd ud-Dīn 'Attār's *Conference of the Birds.*

On pages 44–45 the surgeon's narrative of the operation is blended with material drawn from Howard Carter's 1922–1924 journals, held at Oxford University, describing the discovery and subsequent excavation of Tutankhamen's tomb in the Valley of the Kings, Egypt. www.griffith.ox.ac.uk/gri/4sea1not.html

ACKNOWLEDGMENTS

Many thanks to Martha Rhodes, Ryan Murphy, Hannah Matheson, Trish Marshall, and Rowan Sharp, and everyone at Four Way Books for their contributions to, and belief in, this work.

And deep gratitude, in particular, to those poets, critics, patients, and medical professionals who offered invaluable feedback on earlier drafts: Caleb Carr, Rachel Blau DuPlessis, Joseph Donahue, Norman Finkelstein, John Golfinos, MD, Maeve Kinkead, Dawn McGuire, MD, Nancy Milliken, MD, Alicia Jo Rabins, J. J. Penna, and Abby Wender.

Some of this work appeared, sometimes in slightly different form, in the journals *Salt* and *Middlelost.* I am grateful to these editors for their belief in this work.

About the Author

Elizabeth T. Gray, Jr. is a poet, translator, critic, and corporate consultant. Previous collections of poetry include *Salient* (New Directions, 2020) and *Series | India* (Four Way Books, 2015). *Let Us Believe in the Beginning of the Cold Season* (New Directions, 2022), her translations of Iran's major modern woman poet, Forough Farrokhzad (1937–1962), was a finalist for the 2023 PEN Award for Poetry in Translation. *The Green Sea of Heaven,* a 30th anniversary edition of her translations of Iran's major medieval mystic poet, Háfiz (d. 1389), appeared from Monkfish Publishing in 2024. She currently serves on the Boards of Kimbilio for Black Fiction, the *Beloit Poetry Journal* Foundation, Friends of Writers, and the Abdorrahman Boroumand Center for Human Rights in Iran. She was a founder and managing partner/CEO of Conflict Management, Inc. and Alliance Management Partners, LLC, boutique corporate consulting firms. She holds a BA and JD from Harvard University and an MFA from Warren Wilson and lives in New York City.

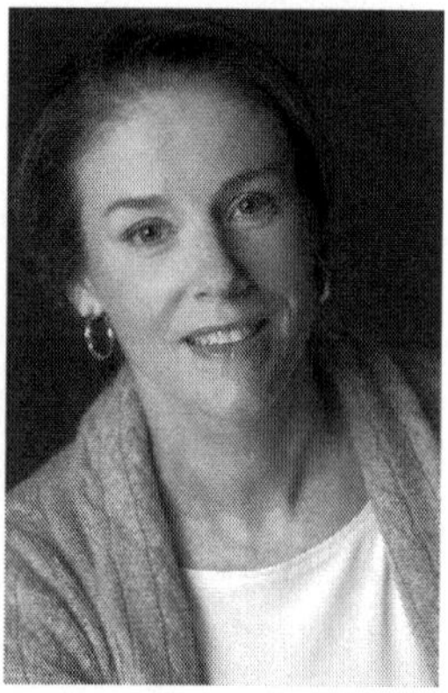

author photo: Susan Johann

We are also grateful to those individuals who participated in our Build a Book Program. They are:

Anonymous (15), Robert Abrams, Debra Allbery, Nancy Allen, Michael Ansara, Kathy Aponick, Jean Ball, Sally Ball, Jill Bialosky, Sophie Cabot Black, Laurel Blossom, Tommye Blount, Karen and David Blumenthal, Jonathan Blunk, Lee Briccetti, Jane Martha Brox, Mary Lou Buschi, Anthony Cappo, Carla and Steven Carlson, Robin Rosen Chang, Liza Charlesworth, Peter Coyote, Elinor Cramer, Kwame Dawes, Michael Anna de Armas, Brian Komei Dempster, Renko and Stuart Dempster, Matthew DeNichilo, Rosalynde Vas Dias, Patrick Donnelly, Charles R. Douthat, Lynn Emanuel, Blas Falconer, Laura Fjeld, Carolyn Forché, Helen Fremont and Donna Thagard, Debra Gitterman, Dorothy Tapper Goldman, Alison Granucci, Naomi Guttman and Jonathan Mead, Jeffrey Harrison, KT Herr, Carlie Hoffman, Melissa Hotchkiss, Thomas and Autumn Howard, Catherine Hoyser, Elizabeth Jackson, Linda Susan Jackson, Jessica Jacobs, Deborah Jonas-Walsh, Jennifer Just, Voki Kalfayan, Maeve Kinkead, Victoria Korth, David Lee and Jamila Trindle, Rodney Terich Leonard, Howard Levy, Owen Lewis and Susan Ennis, Eve Linn, Matthew Lippman, Ralph and Mary Ann Lowen, Maja Lukic, Neal Lulofs, Anthony Lyons, Ricardo Alberto Maldonado, Trish Marshall, Donna Masini, Deborah McAlister, Carol Moldaw, Michael and Nancy Murphy, Kimberly Nunes, Matthew Olzmann and Vievee Francis, Veronica Patterson, Patrick Phillips, Robert Pinsky, Megan Pinto, Kevin Prufer, Anna Duke Reach, Paula Rhodes, Yoana Setzer, James Shalek, Soraya Shalforoosh, Peggy Shinner, Joan Silber, Jane Simon, Debra Spark, Donna Spruijt-Metz, Arlene Stang, Page Hill Starzinger, Catherine Stearns, Yerra Sugarman, Arthur Sze, Laurence Tancredi, Marjorie and Lew Tesser, Peter Turchi, Connie Voisine, Susan Walton, Martha Webster and Robert Fuentes, Calvin Wei, Allison Benis White, Lauren Yaffe, and Rolf Yngve.